Medical Dictionary for Regulatory Activities

MedDRA

copyright@DrRaviNHumbarwadi

www.pro-career.net

Contact:pi.con.publisher@gmail.com

MedDRA

MedDRA: Medical Dictionary for Regulatory Activities.

MedDRA provides standardized medical terminology. It is developed by ICH (international conference of harmonization). This standardization allows seamless sharing of regulatory information globally for medical products. It is used for registration, documentation and safety monitoring of investigational as well as approved drugs.

MedDRA is meant for coding of events, indications for drug use and medical history.

MedDRA can code for symptoms - dizziness, headache, asthenia; diagnosis- transient Ischemic attack, influenza, multiple sclerosis; syndromes- Steven Johnson Syndrome, Fanconi syndrome, Sjogren syndrome and investigation result - hyponatremia, thrombocytopenia, neutropenia.

The MedDRA dictionary is organized by System Organ Class (SOC), which is divided into High-Level Group Terms (HLGT), High-Level Terms (HLT), Preferred Terms (PT) and finally into Lower-Level Terms (LLT).

The MSSO (Maintenance and Support Services Organization), is contracted by ICH to maintain, develop and distribute MedDRA. MedDRA usage is free for regulators, health care providers and academics.

However license to use MedDRA is granted to companies only on a paid subscriptions basis. This payment is calculated taking into account the annual turnover of companies.

Under the governance of the ICH MedDRA Management Board, MedDRA is updated to meet the needs of regulatory authority and keep up with advances in medical science.

MedDRA has transitioned from version 1 to current version. The LLT has more than seventy eight thousand terms. This gives more options for each code so that the coder can choose the most appropriate option.

To facilitate its correct use, free training is offered and MedDRA is also made available in several languages – Chinese, Czech, Dutch, French, German, Hungarian, Italian, Japanese, Portuguese and Spanish.

The current ICH M1 Points to Consider Working Group develops and maintains two documents on the use of MedDRA.

A. Data entry
B. Data retrieval.

The data entry document is for coding purpose and the data retrieval document aids analysis. The data retrieval document includes guidance on the use of Standardised MedDRA Queries (SMQs). The SMQ is an efficient tool used in assessment of safety signal detection. Both, the coding as well as the data retrieval documents are generally updated twice a year, and with every MedDRA release.

Collaboration between ICH and WHO: MedDRA is fully implemented in the WHO global safety database allowing entry and retrieval of information not only through WHO-ART but also through MedDRA.

The MSSO releases updated MedDRA versions twice a year - in March and September. The March release is the main release and contains changes at all levels.

RELATIONSHIP BETWEEN LLT AND PT.

PT	A single medical concept.
LLT	A sub-type, lexican variant or synonym of a preferred term.

1. Sub-type: The LLT can be a sub-type of the PT.

    PT - Limb paresis
    LLT - Transient paresis of limb
    Here the LLT is more specific and describes the paresis as transient.

    PT - Influenza
    LLT - Influenza B virus infection
    Here the LLT describes the type of influenza virus.

    The LLT may specify the anatomical site of the event (ex: generalized) , the type of the infection (B virus) or the nature of the event (ex: transient) . In the sub-type the LLT has more details than the PT.

2. Lexical variants: The terms in the LLT and PT vary. The variation is due to jumbling of word order in and use of abbreviations in the LLT.

A. Jumbled Word order

   PT - Blood pressure increased
   LLT- Pressure blood increased

B. Abbreviations

   PT - Complete Blood Count
   LLT - CBC

3. Synonyms: Different terms for the same disease. PT is a technical (medical) term.

   PT - Asthma
   LLT - Asthma like condition

   PT - Angina pectoris
   LLT - Chest pain-cardiac

Capitalisation is used for the first letter of each term, proper names and abbreviations

Abbreviations are at the LLT level only.

Natural word order is maintained at the PT level. For instance you may find LLT pressure blood increased. But the PT will be Blood pressure increased.

Examples of Event Coding

Example 1.

I have been taking the suspect drug since 3 years. Since six months I have been admitted to the hospital for Chron's flare.

Search: Input – Chron

Options that could appear in the MeDRA dictionary –

Chron's disease

Chron's aggravated

The appropriate code in this case would be Chron's aggravated.

Click on the option and the event will be coded to the appropriate PT, HLT, HLGT and SOC.

Reported verbatim: Chron's Flare

Coded to: Chron's Aggravated.

Example 2.

I was on the suspect drug since middle of May in 2005. In December 2009 I was diagnosed with Diabetes Mellitus.

Search Input: Diabetes Mellitus

The options that may appear in the MedDRA dictionary may include:

Type 1 Diabetes Mellitus

Type 2 Diabetes Mellitus

Diabetes Mellitus

Juvenile Diabetes Mellitus

The appropriate option in this case would be Diabetes Mellitus. We cannot choose type 1 or type 2 since it is not specified in the source document whether it is type 1 or type 2.

In this example you can also choose the autocode option.

The autocode option can be used when the reported terms are highly specific such as dizziness, malaise, hypertension, asthma, Diabetes Mellitus, Parkinson's disease etc.

When you have terms such as 'weakness of limbs associated with fatigue it is not possible to autocode the reported verbatim.'

In case you are not sure or the term does not get autocoded you can choose the manual (interactive) coding option which will throw up a list of options and you will have to choose the most appropriate option.

Example 3

I was on the suspect drug for just a few weeks when I started experiencing pain in the eye and upper limb.

The reported event is: Pain in the eye and upper limb.

In such a scenario it is better to split the term to

Pain in the eye

Pain in the upper limb.

This can then be coded to

Orbital pain

Upper limb Pain

Example 4

A couple of days after taking the suspect drug my cousin had nausea, vomiting, and abdominal pain. The physician diagnosed gastroenteritis.

This is just the opposite of the earlier example.

Here we can just code to gastroenteritis since nausea, vomiting, abdominal pain has been diagnosed as gasttroenteritis.

Example 5

SOC

Blood and Lymphatic System Disorders

HLGT

White Blood Cell Disorders

HLT

Neutropenias

PT

Neutropenia

LLT

Neutropenia / Neutropenia aggravated

Example 6

SOC

Renal and Urinary disorders

HLGT

Urolithiasis

HLT

Urinary Tract Lithiasis (excl renal)

PT

Calculus Urinary

LLT

Calculus urinary

SYSTEM ORGAN CLASSES
- Blood and lymphatic system disorders
- Cardiac disorders
- Congenital, familial and genetic disorders
- labyrinth disorders
- Musculoskeletal and connective tissue disorders
- Neoplasms benign, malignant and unspecified (incl cysts and polyps)
- Endocrine disorders
- Eye disorders
- Gastrointestinal disorders
- Nervous system disorders
- Pregnancy, puerperium and perinatal conditions
- General disorders and administration site conditions
- Hepatobiliary disorders
- Psychiatric disorders
- Renal and urinary disorders
- Reproductive system and breast disorders
- Immune system disorders
- Respiratory, thoracic and mediastinal disorders
- Infections and infestations
- Injury, poisoning and procedural complications
- Skin and subcutaneous tissue disorders
- Social circumstances
- Surgical and medical procedures
- Investigations
- Metabolism and nutrition disorders
- Vascular disorders

MedDRA Hierarchy (Version 21)

System Organ Class (SOC)	27
High Level Group Term (HLGT)	337
High Level Term (HLT)	1737
Preferred Term (PT)	23088
Lowest Level Term (LLT)	78808

MedDRA CODING: A PERSPECTIVE

- Lowest Level Term that most accurately reflects the reported verbatim information should be selected.
- Be specific.
- Avoid soft coding.
- For lab test results take into consideration absence or presence of units.
- Select terms for device-related events, product quality issues, medication errors, medical and social history, investigations and indications. There are many options available to code to the accurate term. Use the search option and familiarize yourselves with the different terms available.
- If there is no exact match in MedDRA, use medical judgment to match an existing term (closest possible match) that adequately represents the reported verbatim.
- If diagnosis is reported along with the signs and symptoms, the preferred option is to code for diagnosis only.

FINAL DIAGNOSIS

Diagnosis along with its characteristic signs symptoms is provided.
Preferred Coding: Diagnosis only.

Example: Pneumonia with fever and cough.
Preferred Coding: Pneumonia.

This is because we know that fever and cough are symptoms of pneumonia.

PROVISIONAL DIAGNOSIS

Provisional diagnosis along with signs and symptoms is provided.
Preferred Coding: Provisional diagnosis plus the signs and symptoms have to be coded.

Example: Possibly a drug allergy with dyspnea and low blood pressure
Preferred Coding: Drug allergy
                                Dyspnea
                                Low blood pressure

SYMPTOMS ONLY

Only symptoms are provided.
Preferred Coding: Code all the reported symptoms.

Example: The patient had fever and cough. Diagnosis was pending.

Preferred Coding: Fever
        Cough

BE SPECIFIC

Being specific is important.

Example: The patient had - paresis of upper limb.
Code To: Upper limb paresis and not just to paresis.

Example: Stress due to work.
Code To: Stress at work and not just to Stress.

Use the search option in MedDRA to select the most specific code.

AVOID SOFT CODING

Coding to a less severe medical condition is termed as soft coding. This has to be avoided.

Example: "End stage renal failure" coded as "Renal impairment"

While there is renal impairment it does not convey that the patient has progressed to end stage renal failure. An inappropriate coding is a wrong coding.

COMBINATION TERMS

Use combination terms whenever available.

Example: Cardiomyopathy due to diabetes
Code To: Diabetic cardiomyopathy

SPLIT TERMS

Split terms when it describes two possible codes.

Example: Pruritic generalized rash
Code To: Generalized rash
       Pruritic rash

LACK OF EFFICACY

Example: The drug did not work
Code To: Lack of drug effect

Example: Patient took the drug for several weeks. Now the drug is not working as it used to.
Code To: Drug effect decreased

UNCLEAR TERMINOLOGY

The source document has thin details and no clarity.

Example: Became pink
Code to: Unevaluable event

"Bacame pink" is vague. It could be that the patient became pink, skin turned pink, possibly an erythema or the syrup color turned pink. Some symptom has been reported but when it could mean so many possibilities it becomes an unevaluable event.

Example: Patient had a problem with his liver
Code To: Liver disorder

Example: Patient had a medical condition and went for investigations
Code To: Ill-defined disorder

This is a general statement. Possibly the reporter had only this information at the time of reporting.

MEDICATION ERRORS

Example: Last week the patient missed taking a dose
Code To: Drug dose omission

Example: Patient received an overdose of medicine
Code To: Drug overdose

Example: Patient with G6PD deficiency is prescribed a drug that is contraindicated in this condition.
Code To: Labeled drug-disease interaction medication error.

These are medication errors without any associated events. So just code to the reported verbatim.

MEDICATION ERRORS WITH ADVERSE EVENTS

Example: Patient was administered wrong drug and experienced dyspnea
Code To: Wrong drug administered
       Dyspnea

Example: Because of similar sounding drug names, the patient took the wrong drug and developed edema
Code To: Drug name confusion
       Wrong drug administered
       Edema

Example: There was a prescription error and the patient had diplopia
Code To: Drug prescribing error
          Diplopia

Prescription errors – When doctor's do not follow the recommendations and cross the maximum or minimum dose or frequency when prescribing a drug.

The other prescription errors are:

Drug dose prescribing error
Drug dosage form prescribing error
Drug dose schedule prescribing error
Drug route prescribing error

As you can see in addition to the events that have occurred it is also mandatory to capture and code the associated medication errors. Note that there are various types of medication errors and these have to be identified and coded appropriately.

INVESTIGATION RESULT CODING

Example: Hb 8 g/dl
Code To: Haemoglobin low

Units are given and so we can be sure that the result is low

Example: Calcium 3.3
Code To: Blood calcium abnormal

The calcium normal values are 8.5 to 10.5 mg/dL and also 2.12 to 2.62 mmol/L.
This could be high or low calcium depending on the units. Since units are not provided code to calcium abnormal.

WHO Drug Dictionary (WHO DD)

The WHO Drug Dictionary is a classification of medicines by the WHO Program for International Drug Monitoring. It is managed by the Uppsala Monitoring Centre (UMC).

It is used by sponsors, clinical research organizations and regulatory authorities for identification and coding of drugs in spontaneous and clinical trial reports.

The new WHO Drug Dictionary Enhanced is the result of collaboration of UMC with IMS Health. It contains data from the WHO Drug Dictionary and also from IMS Health and has been developed using formats which are similar to those in the WHO Drug Dictionary.

The WHO Drug Dictionary Enhanced contains the most number of product names and is the most comprehensive drug product information. Many suspect, concomitant or past drugs can easily have a direct match and this in turn can lead to increased accuracy and speed of drug coding.

Brand drugs need to be input and coded to its generic using the WHO-DD. Generics have to coded as reported.

PHARMACOVIGILANCE

NARRATIVE WRITING

1. Introduction

2. ICH Guidelines

3. Special Scenarios

    - Licensee partner
    - Off label
    - Clinical trial reports
    - Pregnancy cases
    - Regulatory authority
    - Voice calls

Narrative Writing

Case narrative writing is an important part of pharmacovigilance and patient safety. The quality of the report is key for evaluating a potential link between the product and adverse events.

Patient narratives are written for serious adverse events (SAEs), adverse events (AEs) of special clinical interest, important medical events and fatal (death) cases.

Patient narratives are relevant for reporting both clinical trials and post marketing studies. It forms an important component of clinical study reports (CSRs) and pharmacovigilance activities (e.g. post marketing safety reports).

Specifically, narratives should include:

• Patient identifier

• Age and sex of patient; ethnicity; general clinical condition of patient

• Disease being treated with duration (of current episode) of illness

• Relevant coexisting/previous illnesses with details of occurrence/duration

• Relevant concomitant/previous medication with details of dosage

• Test drug administered, including dose, if this varied among patients, and length of time administered.

As per International Conference on Harmonisation (ICH) E3 (Section 12.3.2), a patient narrative should describe:

- An indication of study drug administration
- The nature, intensity and outcome of the event
- The clinical course leading to the event
- Relevant laboratory measures
- Action taken with the study drug (and timing) in relation to the event
- Treatment or intervention
- Post mortem findings (if applicable)
- Investigator's and Sponsor's (if appropriate) opinion on causality

ICSR Narrative Writing

1. Lead sentence should define type of report, day 0, source of report

2. Patient details: age, ethnicity, gender and country

3. Concurrent medical condition, concomitant drugs and past drugs

4. Suspect drug details: indication, dosage, start and stop date

5. Event details

6. Treatment provided for event

7. Event outcome

8. Causality between event and suspect drug

Sample 1: Spontaneous report was received from Licensee Partner

This spontaneous case was received by licensee partner name (licensee number) on ----------- (day 0) and was forwarded to manufacturer on --------- (date received).

This case concerns 50-year-old Caucasian female patient from --------- (country).

Medical history included: hypertension, diabetes and family history of cancer, surgical procedures includes: hysterectomy. Social history includes: smoking. Concomitant medications included: metformin, paracetamol, methotrexate and nifedipine, all used for unknown indications. Past drug history included: ------- medications.

On 06-Aug-2009, the patient initiated therapy with XYZ drug, formulation, at dose of 10 mg, for indication.

On 09-Feb-2010, the patient experienced pneumonia and was hospitalized. The patient was treated with azithromycin.

On an unknown date in 2010 the event resolved and the patient was discharged on 03-Mar-2010.

At the time of this report, the outcome of event was resolved. Therapy status with XYZ was unknown.

The reporter did not provide causality of event for treatment with XYZ drug.

Note

- Licensee partner cases require minimal changes.
- Licensee partners tend to send ready cases

Sample 2: Case with an Off Label use of drug based on frequency (or indication/ dose/ population).

This spontaneous case was received by from a consumer.

This case concerns an off label use of suspect drug for frequency as per local labeling of United States of America.

This case concerned a 71 year old female patient from United States of America.

The patient's medical history included shellfish allergy, hypothyroidism, and osteoporosis.

The patient's previously reported events included cardiac stent placement in Jul-2008.

On 07-Aug-2003, the patient started treatment with suspect drug in the form of 500 mg/ml oral solution at a total nightly dose of 7.5 gram (two equal doses) for cataplexy. The batch number and expiry date were not reported.

On an unknown date, in Apr-2015, the reporter stated that she did not take her medication for several days in April because a lump was found in her breast (medically significant) and she had to go for several tests.

The reporter also stated that she did not take most of her second doses because she had to drive early in the morning.

The reporter stated that she had the lump and the nodes removed on Monday night and will have a follow-up on 19-May-2015.

It was unknown if the patient continued treatment with minocycline. The outcome of the events was not reported.

Company reference number: BL-2015-012631

Sample: Clinical trial reports

1. If it is interventional study: It is important to mention if pre-treatment case or post-treatment case.

2. Mention investigator causality for all the reported events

3. Events are already picked by the investigator

4. Better structured source makes case processing, event picking and narrative writing easier.

Clinical Trial Case Narrative

This study interventional report was received by Manufacturer on day 0 from an investigator.

This case concerns 25-year-old Hispanic male patient who was enrolled in particular study.

Medical history included: atrial fibrillation, hypertension, stroke and type I diabetes. Concomitant medications included: aspirin, metformin and nuvigil.

On 06-Mar-2015, the patient received the first dose of study drug at 200 mg, every 2 weeks via oral route.

On an unknown date in Mar-2015, the patient had urinary tract infection and had been put on Trimethoprim.

Mention all related lab test and results.

At the time of report, treatment with study drug was ongoing. The Outcome of the event was not resolved.

The investigator assessed the causality for the event as related to the study drug

Sample: Pregnancy Case

1. If the outcome of pregnancy is known then it is a retrospective pregnancy

2. If outcome of pregnancy is unknown that is prospective pregnancy

3. Mention type of pregnancy – vaginal, caesarean

4. Duration of gestation and whether premature or tem delivery

5. Medical history or BOH- bad obstetric history

6. APGAR score and status of fetus including height and weight

7. Status of breast feeding

Case 1

This prospective pregnancy spontaneous case was received by manufacturer on day 0 from a consumer.

This case concerns 30-year-old female patient from United Kingdom who received XYZ drug, formulation, for narcolepsy.

Medical history included: hyperlipidaemia, thyroid problems, sleep apnea and chronic pain.

In Apr-2013, the patient initiated therapy with XYZ at dose og 2.5 mg, twice daily via oral route. From an unknown date in 2013, the XYZ dose was changed to 3 mg, twice daily.

The patient's reported last menstrual period was on 09-Sep-2013 (pregnancy). Estimated due date of delivery was 16-Jun-2014

On an unknown date in 2013, the patient discontinued XYZ due to pregnancy.

At the time of this report, therapy with XYZ was discontinued.

Case 2

This retrospective pregnancy study case was received by manufacturer on 20-Apr-2015 from a healthcare professional via BUPA healthcare/ patient support program

This case concerns an adult female patient from United Kingdom.

Medical history included: spontaneous abortion.

On 04-Jan-2014, the patient became pregnant.

In Sep-2014, the patient initiated treatment with ABC drug, solution for injection, at dose of 40 mg, every two weeks for rheumatoid arthritis via subcutaneous route. The baby was exposed via transplacental route.

On 11-Oct-2014, the mother delivered a healthy baby of weight 3120 gm, 14 cm of Apgar score 9/9 via C-section.

From an unknown date, the patient was breastfed.

At the time of this report, the outcome of C-Section was unknown. Therapy with ABC was ongoing.

Sample: Case from Regulatory Authority

For example MHRA

Lead sentence should mention authority name.

This spontaneous regulatory authority case was received by manufacturer on day 0 from a consumer/physician/healthcare professional via MHRA (Authority No.)

Sample: Case via Voice Call

This spontaneous case was received by Pharmy from a male patient who had been on valproate sodium in 2014. Voice message and a phone call received on 04-May-2015 from the United States.

www.pro-career.net

www.xillaclub.com

Pro-career.net

1. Pharmacovigilance

2. Clinical Research

3. PV Database

4. Pharmacoepidemiology

5. Drug Safety Mega Book

www.pro-career.net

The Online Library

Shape Your Career

www.xillaclub.com

Audio

Reshape Your Life

www.ingramcontent.com/pod-product-compliance
Lightning Source LLC
Chambersburg PA
CBHW030517220526
45464CB00006B/2839